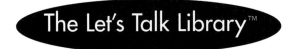

Let's Talk About Stuttering

Susan Kent

The Rosen Publishing Group's
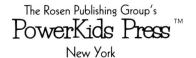
PowerKids Press™
New York

For Marty Jezer and Paul Johnson

Published in 2000 by The Rosen Publishing Group, Inc.
29 East 21st Street, New York, NY 10010

First Edition

Book design: Erin McKenna

Photo Illustrations on pp. 4, 7, 11, 12, 15, 16, 19, 20 by Thaddeus Harden; p.8 © Everett Collection,Inc.

Kent, Susan, 1942—
    Let's talk about stuttering / by Susan Kent.
        p.   cm. — (The Let's talk library)
    Includes index.
    Summary: Discusses stuttering, the embarrassment it may cause, and the possibility of self-esteem for those with this condition.
    ISBN 0-8239-5423-4 (lib. bdg.)
    1. Stuttering—Juvenile literature. [1. Stuttering.] I. Title. II. Series.
RC424.K43 1999
616.85'54—dc21   98-50160
                                                                                  CIP
                                                                                  AC

Manufactured in the United States of America

Table of Contents

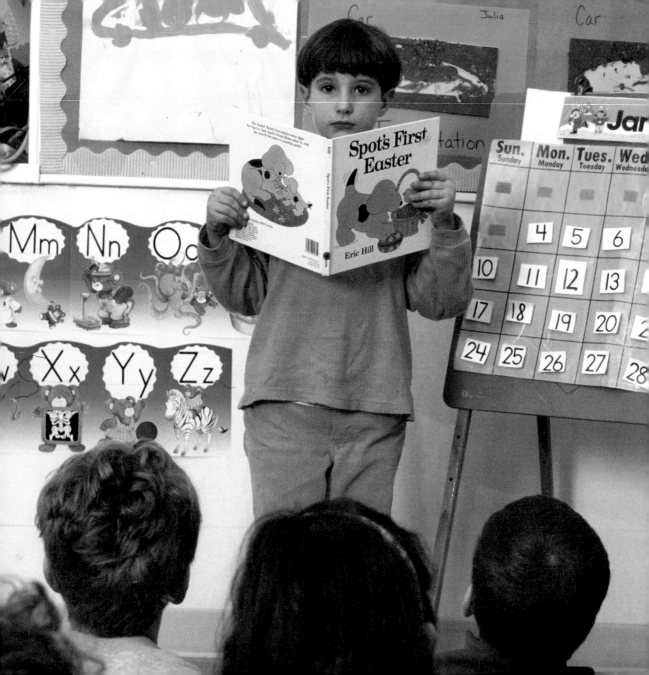

Brandon

Brandon's class goes to the library to pick out books for their book reports. Brandon chooses one about a boy and his dog. The dog on the cover looks just like Brandon's dog, Freckles. Brandon loves the book and has fun writing his report. His teacher stamps a smiley face on his paper.

Now his teacher has asked him to read the book to the whole class. Brandon doesn't want to read out loud because he **stutters**. He is worried he will not be able to say the words clearly.

◀ *Sometimes, people who stutter find it hard to speak in front of others.*

What Is Stuttering?

Stuttering is blocked, "bumpy," or broken speech. It is also sometimes called stammering. If you stutter, it means you have trouble speaking.

You may repeat the first part of a word, such as d-d-d-daddy or da-da-da-daddy, or hold onto one sound for an extra long time, such as mmmm-mommy or c-aaaaa-t. Maybe you use a different vowel, such as seh-seh-sister. Sometimes you may make no sound at all, or have trouble getting sounds out.

If you stutter, sometimes you might twist your face or jerk your head when you try to get words out. ▶

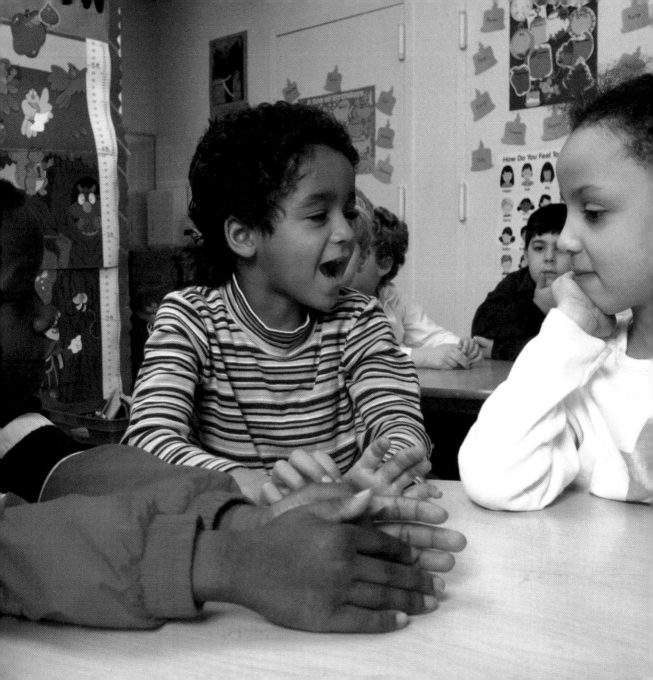

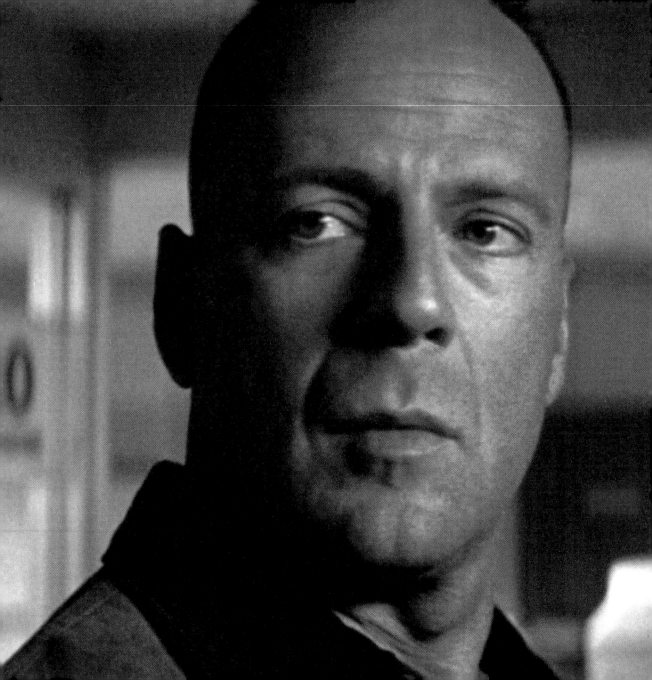

Who Stutters?

If you stutter, you are not alone. About three million people stutter. In fact, everyone has trouble speaking sometimes, even your parents and teachers. Listen closely and you'll hear them. Stuttering can get better over time. Many children stutter but then grow out of it. Of those who continue to stutter, more are boys than girls.

People who stutter are not different from other people. They are just as smart, as healthy, and as much fun to be with.

◀ *Lots of people stutter, even famous movie stars like Bruce Willis.*

What Makes Someone Stutter?

No one knows the cause of stuttering, or why more boys stutter than girls. Sometimes more than one person in a family stutters.

Stuttering often happens when you have strong feelings, like anger or fear, but it is not caused by these feelings. It is also not caused by anything people do to you. Although no one knows what causes stuttering, there is one important thing that we do know. Stuttering is not anyone's fault—not yours and not your parents'.

This boy doesn't stutter all the time, but he often stutters when he is nervous or upset. ▶

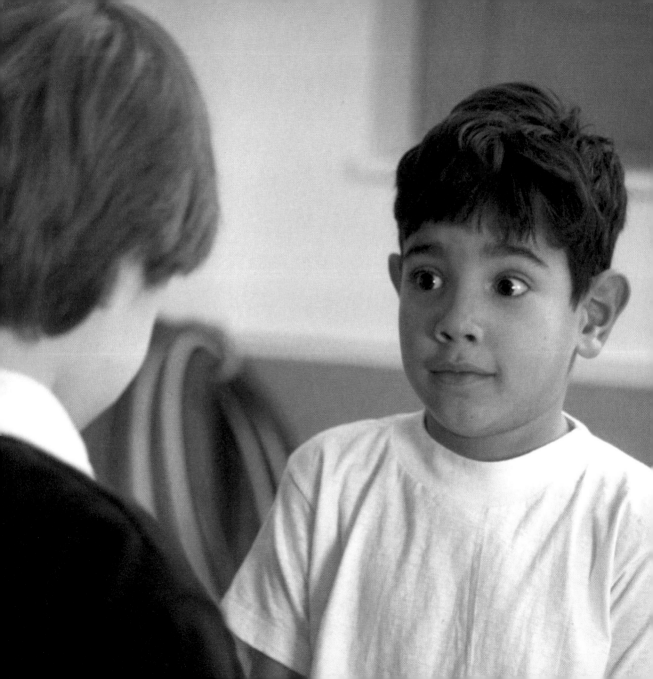

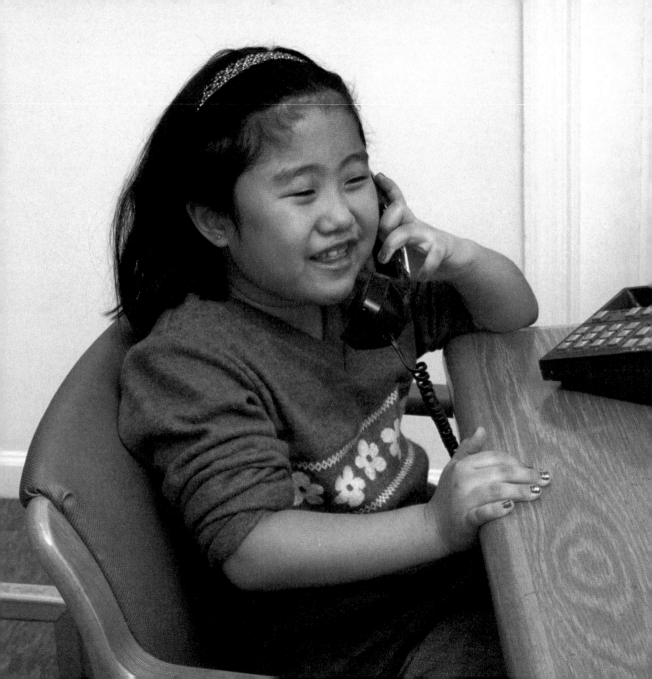

When Do You Stutter?

People stutter most when they are nervous, tired, excited, or upset. You might also stutter when you first wake up or when you talk on the telephone. Your stuttering can get worse when you try hardest to hide it. This can be very **frustrating**.

No one stutters all the time. You probably do not stutter when you are very calm, or when you sing, whisper, or talk to animals. Worrying about when you will stutter can make you feel **anxious**.

◀ *People stutter at different times. Some people stutter when they talk on the telephone.*

Cassie

Cassie is tired of being teased about her stuttering. She tells her parents, and together they plan what to do about it.

The next day, Cassie is jumping rope with her friends when Zoe calls out, "C-c-c-c-cassie!" Cassie tries ignoring her, but that doesn't stop her. Zoe comes closer and says, "C-c-c-cassie, c-c-c-cat, g-got your t-t-t-tongue?" Cassie then tries humor. She says to Zoe, "Do you st-t-tutter, t-t-too, or are you ju-just rude?" Everyone laughs, and, for once, Zoe has nothing to say.

Cassie feels happy that she got Zoe to stop teasing her about her stuttering. ▶

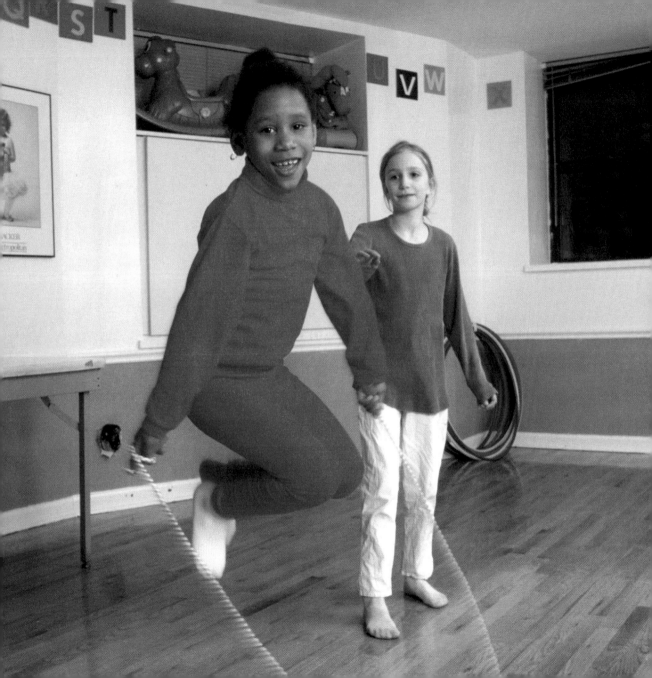

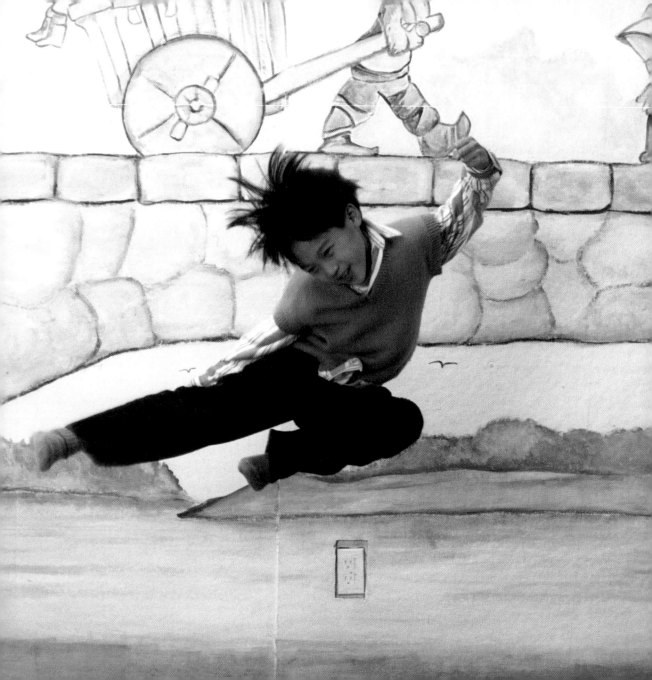

Your Feelings About Stuttering

If you stutter, you might sometimes feel bad about yourself. When you trip over words, you feel **embarrassed**. When you are teased, your feelings get hurt. You might start to think that because you have trouble speaking, you can't do anything right, but that's not true.

Stuttering is something you do. It is not who you are. You are a terrific person! You can stutter and still do whatever you want. You can be a ballplayer, a singer, a dancer, or even an actor.

◀ *This boy doesn't let his stuttering get in the way of practicing his karate moves!*

Getting Help

If your stuttering bothers you, **therapists** called **speech-language pathologists** can help. They teach you how to breathe smoothly and evenly, and how to **relax** your lips, jaw, tongue, and throat when you speak. They play games with you that can help improve your stuttering. You might build with blocks or blow bubbles. You and your therapist might play cards or lotto, and take turns talking. You learn to do things the slow-and-easy way rather than the fast-and-hard way.

Speech pathologists are fun to visit. They help you feel good about yourself and your speech. ▶

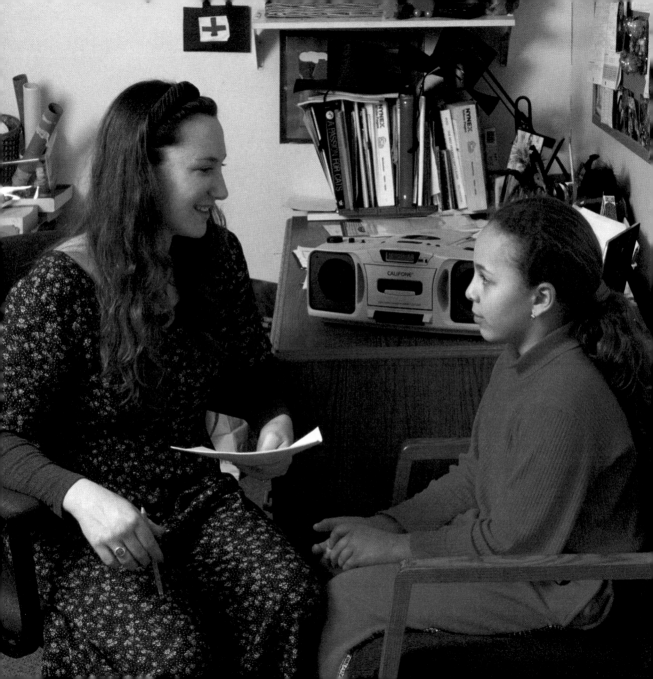

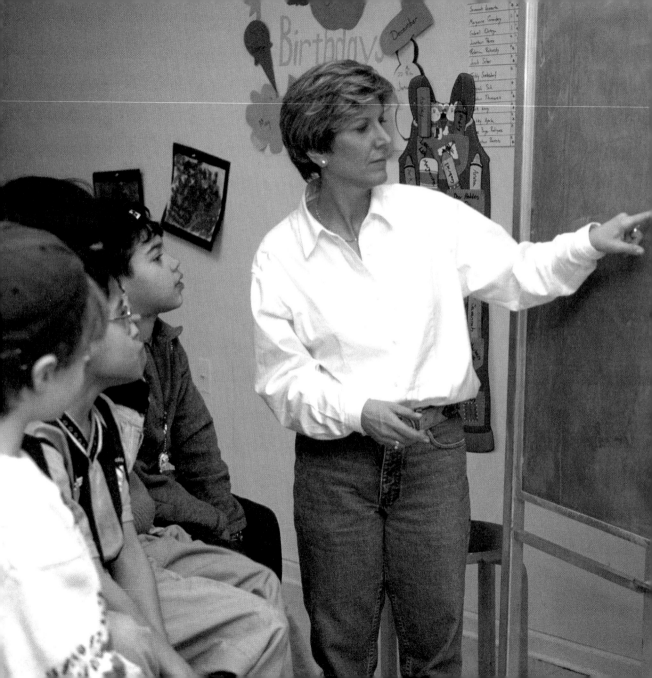

Felipe

Felipe's speech therapist comes to his classroom. She talks about stuttering. She reminds the class that although he stutters, Felipe is a good singer and a fast runner. She asks some students to talk into a machine that makes them sound like they stutter. After his classmates try it, they tell Felipe they now have a better understanding of how he feels. Jimmy says he is sorry for teasing Felipe. Felipe is happy because he doesn't have to try to hide his stuttering anymore. He feels better about his stuttering and about himself.

◀ *This speech pathologist talks to a class about stuttering. She helps them understand what it might be like to stutter.*

When Friends Stutter

What should you do when friends stutter? First, never tease them! Try hard not to look away. Don't hurry your friends. Don't interrupt them or finish their sentences for them. Take the time to listen to what your friends are saying. Though they speak slowly, they still have important things to say. Let them know that you are glad they are your friends and that they are great people!

If you would like more information about stuttering, you can write to:

FRIENDS, Association of Young People Who Stutter
1220 Rosita Road
Pacifica, CA 94044-4223

Glossary

anxious (AYNK-shus) Uneasy or worried.

embarrassed (im-BAYR-ist) Feeling uncomfortable or ashamed.

frustrating (FRUS-tray-ting) When not being able to change a situation makes you feel angry or sad.

relax (ree-LAKS) To feel loose and let go of stiffness, tension, or worry.

speech-language pathologist (SPEECH–LANG-gwij pah-THAH-luh-jist) Someone who helps people who have problems speaking.

stutter (STUH-tur) To speak with pauses or blocks and to repeat sounds.

therapist (THER-uh-pist) A person who helps someone when they are having a hard time with something.

Index